Weight Loss Tips for the Struggling Dieter

How to Lose Weight without the Stress

By: Wendy Chin

TABLE OF CONTENTS

Wendy Chin
PUBLISHERS NOTES

Speedy Publishing LLC

40 E. Main St., #1156

Newark, DE 19711

www.speedypublishing.co

Cover Artwork: 24 Hr. Designs Ltd.

Editing: Speedy Publishing LLC

Book design: Speedy Publishing LLC

ISBN:

This is a reprint book.

DISCLAIMER

This publication is intended to provide helpful and informative material. It is not intended to diagnose, treat, cure, or prevent any health problem or condition, nor is intended to replace the advice of a physician. No action should be taken solely on the contents of this book. Always consult your physician or qualified health-care professional on any matters regarding your health and before adopting any suggestions in this book or drawing inferences from it.

The author and publisher specifically disclaim all responsibility for any liability, loss or risk, personal or otherwise, which is incurred as a consequence, directly or indirectly, from the use or application of any contents of this book.

Any and all product names referenced within this book are the trademarks of their respective owners. None of these owners have sponsored, authorized, endorsed, or approved this book.

Always read all information provided by the manufacturers' product labels before using their products. The author and publisher are not responsible for claims made by manufacturers.

DEDICATION

This book is dedicated to my family members who helped me to lose the excess weight. A support group is essential to success.

INTRODUCTION

I tried to lose weight for many years unsuccessfully. I can't even count how many diets I tried, and all of them failed for one reason or another.

That's not to say I didn't lose weight. There were a few programs that actually helped me to shed a few pounds, but because of how complicated and restricted the programs were, I always fell off the weight loss wagon, and gained all of my weight back – plus some.

I'm sure you've been there, trying your hardest to lose weight and willing to do just about anything to reach your goals only to struggle to either lose the weight or come all that way, only to struggle to keep it off.

The majority of diet plans make it hard on us, because unless we have the self-discipline to closely follow and monitor a specific routine, we will ultimately lose our way, out of frustration, confusion or simply being overwhelmed.

And if we had the discipline needed, we wouldn't be overweight in the first place!

Throughout the years, I have tried most of the popular weight loss programs on the market, including:

- ❖ The Atkins Diet – I got tired of meat very quickly.
- ❖ The low fat diet – I actually gained weight with this one!
- ❖ The low calorie diet – I was always hungry, and tired.
- ❖ The cabbage soup diet – I got bored quickly.
- ❖ The negative calorie diet – Very difficult to follow and maintain.
- ❖ The grapefruit diet – Impossible to stay on track!

- ❖ Weight Watchers – Frustrating counting points!
- ❖ Jenny Craig – Too costly, and complicated.
- ❖ Slim Fast – I was always hungry and tired.
- ❖ NutriSystem – While I lost some weight, it was expensive to maintain.

There were countless other programs that I suffered through, desperately hoping that one would work. Just one.

One Magic System

But nothing gave me a long term system that I could stick to, and I was close to giving up, resolving to the idea that I would always be overweight and that there was little I could do about it.

Sure, some of these programs would point me in the right direction, but I always ended up so confused with counting calories, or worrying about the "right" foods to eat that I would get so overwhelmed that the EASY thing to do was just give up. And I did. Many, many times.

But I was wrong in the way that I was approaching my weight loss goal and in many cases, I was making things harder than they really had to be.

We CAN make changes that WILL produce results, and we CAN follow a system that WILL be easy to stick to, and best of all, we can still lose weight despite our lifestyles, or how busy our daily lives are.

What would you say if I told you that you could start losing weight without restricting yourself to bland foods that you absolutely dislike, or without having to spend more than 20 minutes a day working out and being active?

Weight Loss Tips for the Struggling Dieter

It's true! By simplifying our weight loss plan down to the basic elements of what really works in terms of losing and maintaining a healthy weight, we can eliminate any chance of sabotaging ourselves or ending up confused and frustrated.

After all, the main reason why we give up on diets or weight loss systems is because they are usually so incredibly time consuming that we can't possibly find time in our daily lives to fit it all in.

Or worse, the diet plans or foods that we are allowed to eat are so limiting and restricted, that we eventually give up, go on a binge caving into the cravings.

We love food. We love the taste, the texture and the many different kinds available. We should be able to enjoy our meals without worrying that we will make a mistake, or that we will destroy our chances of keeping the weight off, once we achieve our goals.

In all honesty, we do NOT have to worry about all of that.

Just by making small changes to our daily lives, our routines and the way that we eat (as well as how much we eat), we can start losing weight without having to sweat the small stuff.

If we want a treat, we have it on our "Cheat Day". If we are craving ice cream or chocolate, we reward ourselves once a week.

A healthy and reasonable weight loss plan involves moderation, not restriction, because we all know that if we're restricted in any way, we ARE going to fail.

We need the freedom to make mistakes without feeling guilty, to learn as we go, and ultimately, to learn how to live healthier, happier lives by being conscious about the decisions we make and understanding how to make better ones.

The primary goals of this plan are to:

- ❖ Increase your metabolism.
- ❖ Help you lose weight without being hungry.
- ❖ Teach you how to eat for the rest of your life.

We need to boost up your metabolism so you will lose weight faster, even while eating plenty of food.

We need to keep you happy and motivated so you can stay on track, even during "rough patches" (and there will be a few along the way) and most importantly, we need to understand how to keep the weight off so we don't ever return to this place in our lives again.

So say goodbye to diet plans. From today forward, we are making a long-term commitment to living a healthier life without restrictions or limits!

HOW TO UNDERSTAND YOUR BODY

One of the biggest problems that we face when struggling to lose weight is that we rarely listen to our bodies, and what it is trying to tell us.

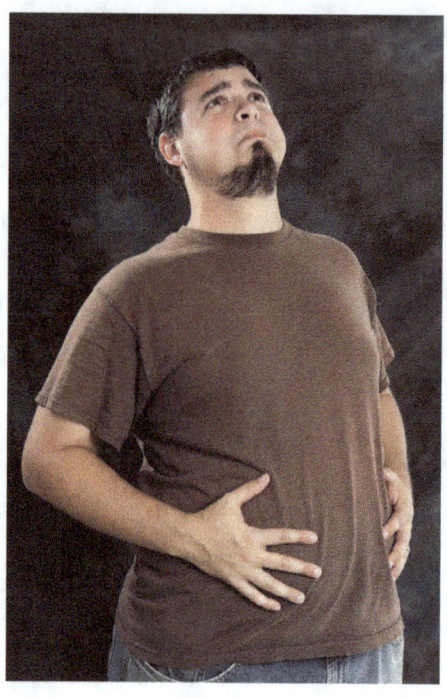

Over the years, through self-indulgence and not paying attention to what we are putting INTO our bodies and how it actually affects us, we lose our internal ability to judge what we really need to be eating. Thankfully, it's very easy to train yourself to listen to your body; it just takes a little bit of practice.

One of the best things about listening to your body is that you won't have to feel deprived or hungry. When you eat what your body is craving, you naturally eat less, or you eat more, but healthier foods that nourish your body and give you the energy and mental clarity that you need.

You see, when you're eating all of that junk food that is nutritionally lacking, your body needs to continue to signal to you that you're hungry so you will eat more and more. If it never gets enough of the nutrients it needs, it will keep you perpetually hungry!

Once you start listening to your body and giving it what it needs, you'll find yourself naturally losing weight. Your body won't hold on to that extra fat anymore, because it won't think its starving.

And you won't feel deprived because you'll still be able to eat many of the foods you love!

Your body is a remarkable instrument. It is precisely calibrated to work at maximum efficiency naturally. If you take care of it properly, it will continue to run at peak efficiency. However, if you abuse it and neglect it, it will begin to wear down quickly.

Since most of us grow up eating a lot of junk foods like candy, cookies, cake, pizza, and potato chips, our bodies are never given enough of the different nutrients it needs. Those foods are empty calories that cause us to gain weight, but don't actually provide us with any vitamins or minerals.

Since our bodies don't get enough nutrients, they continually crave more and more food. Our bodies keep telling us to consume more, because we think we are starving! Surely we must not be taking in enough food if we aren't getting those nutrients, right?

In the wild that would rarely happen except in times of famine. Animals instinctively know what types of foods they should consume, how much, and when. They don't overeat, because they get the right nutrients.

The only time animals in the wild have trouble getting enough of the right nutrients is during times of famine, when their food supply is threatened.

During times of famine, a body's normal reaction is to conserve energy. This is done by putting on weight.

The body stores fat to be converted to energy later when there is no food available.

Additionally, the metabolism slows down in order to keep that weight on as long as possible, so it lasts as long as necessary to keep the body alive during the duration of the famine. This is a natural part of life.

Humans have evolved to eat foods that aren't nutritionally adequate. There are very few nutrients in French fries or a chocolate bar. Even the "healthy" foods we eat are often cooked until most of the vitamins have been destroyed.

In order to learn to listen to your body again, you have to start paying very close attention to the foods you are craving. Usually the body has cravings for certain foods based on nutrients it isn't getting enough of.

For example, a human living in the wild in the wintertime would be without many nutrients for several months. All of the fruits and vegetables would either be long stored-away by animals or buried under snow.

During this time, their primary food source would probably be animals. They would probably have to eat mostly fish until the plants began to produce again.

After a while, that human would very likely begin to crave fish, long after there was a good supply of vegetables or fruits. This is because the body builds a preference for the vitamins and minerals found in specific foods, and once your body has experienced the extra energy and vitality that comes from eating healthier foods, your brain and overall system continues to crave those nutrients and proteins.

By breaking down whatever you're craving, you can learn to figure out what it is your body is really looking for. This is the key to finally losing weight!

There is one important thing you should know about cravings. They aren't ALWAYS indicative of your body needing something.

Cravings can also be triggered by:

- ❖ Hormonal changes (pregnancy, premenstrual syndrome)
- ❖ MSG (monosodium glutamate)
- ❖ Food addiction
- ❖ Depression

These are just a few of the issues that can cause cravings. It can be difficult to tell whether a craving is legitimate or not, but if you substitute something similar and you're still experiencing the craving, odds are the craving was not a legitimate health craving.

MSG is one notable cause of cravings. It has been proven to be very addictive, and food manufacturers and restaurants will often put it in their food to make people crave it.

You should avoid eating foods that contain this addictive substance whenever possible. Eating food that contains MSG will only make you crave more of it, and this perpetuates obesity.

MSG has many harmful effects. It has been linked with:

- ❖ Diabetes – It causes the pancreas to produce three times more insulin than normal!
- ❖ Autism
- ❖ ADD and ADHD
- ❖ Alzheimer's Disease
- ❖ Migraines and General Headaches
- ❖ Brain Lesions
- ❖ Obesity
- ❖ Other Degenerative Diseases Like ALS and Parkinson's

MSG and aspartame (the artificial sweetener) belong to a dangerous group of substances known as excitotoxins. These toxins are believed to be responsible for contributing to many of the above conditions and problems.

If you aren't going to avoid MSG and aspartame, your cravings are going to be more difficult to identify properly. You will probably have a lot of "false positives" and you'll likely be craving things your body isn't physically craving.

Wendy Chin

Eating to Energize the Body

Once you've discovered how to listen to what your body wants, it's time to interpret these cravings and give your body what it wants.

If you're craving pizza, it's probably the tomato sauce your body is asking for. In this case, you could try having some healthy tomato soup, some tomato juice, or a nice, fresh tomato salad.

If you are craving something healthy like watermelon or broccoli, by all means indulge! But of course most people tend to crave things that they really love to eat. Maybe watermelon is your favorite food, and if so, that's great. But most people have less healthy favorites like pizza and French fries as their favorites.

Remember, MSG can cause you to crave foods that your body doesn't need.

You have to break away from the addictive cycle, so you should at least cut down on MSG if you don't eliminate it entirely.

I find I crave cheesecake a lot. For a long time I thought maybe I was craving the calcium, but then I realized I don't just crave cheesecake, I crave strawberry cheesecake!

Once I started eating fresh strawberries once a cheesecake craving hit, I rarely craved it anymore. Sometimes I would still want cheesecake after I ate strawberries, which signaled that I just wanted the flavor of cheesecake. I knew that wasn't a real craving, so I had to make the decision to either ignore the craving, or give in and indulge.

The thing is, you CAN give in and indulge from time to time. You just can't go overboard if you want to lose weight. I would have a very small slice of cheesecake, eating slowly and savoring each bite for the longest time possible.

If I was still craving it after that slice, I would wait at least two hours before giving in again, for another very small slice. And each time I had to decide whether to indulge or not. The strength of the craving was the major deciding factor in whether I would indulge.

Life is short. It's too short to deny yourself entirely. Once I realized that, it was easier for me to lose weight. You see, sticking with a diet is really tough when you never get to eat anything you enjoy!

But when you allow yourself treats and indulgences from time to time, it's a lot easier to keep going. You have more of a reason to keep it up.

You remember the four food groups, right? Unless you're relatively young, you were probably taught about the four food groups in school. Supposedly those were the foods we needed to make up a healthy diet.

These days, it's all about the "food pyramid". The USDA has devised a new way of teaching people about the right foods to eat, dividing foods up even further. It contains 6 groups of foods instead of four.

Well, this food pyramid is actually a lot smarter than the original four food groups, because it actually distinguishes fats, oils, and sweets from healthier foods.

Additionally, fruits and vegetables are in two different groups.

The Food Pyramid

Wendy Chin

The largest group is the base of the pyramid. This group contains breads, grains, and other starches (like corn and potatoes). This is the group the USDA believes you should eat the most of.

These grains and starches help give you energy, but they can be loaded with carbohydrates that can raise your blood sugar. It's best to stick with whole grains, and go easy on the really starchy foods like potatoes.

The USDA recommends that adults consume around 6 to 11 servings of grains and starches per day. Be careful to monitor your portion sizes carefully!

A single slice of bread is one serving, but a slice of thick-sliced bread is TWO servings, and a standard 6-inch sub sandwich roll is THREE servings!

The next level of the pyramid contains fruits and vegetables.

Originally fruits and vegetables were in the same food group when it came to the "four food groups", but a distinction needed to be made. You need to eat both fruits AND vegetables in order to have the healthiest possible diet, so the USDA decided to draw a separation between the two.

Ideally, you want to have at least 3-5 servings of vegetables and 204 servings of fruit each day. A typical serving of vegetables is 1 cup raw or 1 cup cooked. A typical fruit serving is 1 small fresh fruit or 1 cup canned fruit.

The next level of the pyramid shows dairy and protein. The dairy section is smaller than the meat section, because you don't need as much milk per day as you do protein.

You should be getting at least 2-3 servings of dairy per day, preferably low-fat or non-fat. This could include things like milk, yogurt, or even low-fat ice cream.

Proteins include meats and seafood, dried beans, eggs, cheese, and peanut butter. Yes, cheese is included in protein rather than dairy.

You want to get 4-6 ounces of protein daily, ideally from low-fat varieties such as most seafoods, egg whites, low-fat cottage cheese, and skinless poultry. Tofu is also a good choice if you like it.

The final group includes fats, sweets, and alcohol. You should keep these to a minimum. Remember, you do need some fat in your diet, but excessive fat can lead to obesity, especially when consumed with excessive amounts of carbohydrates.

You should have a maximum of 1-2 servings from this group per day, especially when trying to lose weight.

It's not easy keeping track of all of these things, so I don't actually worry too much about counting each and every serving and adding it all up during the day.

What I do is I develop menus for the week, and I plan each meal in a specific way. That way I don't have to worry about adding things up, because it all happens quite naturally.

Here's an example of my weekly meal plan:

Breakfast

3 servings grains
1 serving fruit
1 serving protein
1 serving dairy

Wendy Chin
Lunch

4 servings grains
1 serving fruit
2 servings vegetables
1 serving protein
1 serving dairy
1 serving fat (if not at dinner)

Dinner

2 servings grains
1 serving vegetables
2 servings protein
1 serving fat (if not at lunch)

Snack

1 serving fruit

Snack

1 serving vegetables

That's 3 meals and two snacks per day, which might seem like a lot of food when you're dieting, but it's not. You MUST keep eating regularly to keep your metabolism high. If you don't, your weight loss is going to be much slower than you'd like.

As you can see, this gives me each day:

9 servings grains
3 servings fruit
5 servings vegetables
4 servings protein
2 servings dairy

1 serving of fat

This is a good balance. It's right in the middle of the grains, on the low end of protein and dairy, and on the high end of fruits and vegetables. That's what really got me the best weight loss, because fruits and vegetables are obviously lower in fat and calories than meat and dairy, and I stayed right in the middle for grains to give me enough energy without overeating.

This is what a typical menu would look like:

Breakfast

3 servings oatmeal (small bowl)
1 serving applesauce (in the oatmeal)
1-ounce bacon or ham
1 cup non-fat milk (half over the oatmeal)

Lunch

2 sandwiches with:
2 slices whole grain bread each
Lettuce and tomato
3 ounce low-fat turkey on each
1 tbsp. mayonnaise (half on each)
1 apple
1 cup non-fat milk

Dinner

Noodle Stir-Fry with:
2 servings whole wheat pasta
1 cup steamed broccoli
2 ounces grilled chicken
Herbs and 0 calorie seasonings to taste

Wendy Chin

Snack (between breakfast and lunch or lunch and dinner)

1 cup cantaloupe cubes

Snack (between lunch and dinner or after dinner)

1 cup salad with fat-free dressing

As you can see, this keeps you eating all day long, and you get a considerable amount of food each time. If you're hungry, eat! Just be sure you're really hungry.

It can be quite difficult to tell if you're actually hungry or if you are just bored or depressed and want to eat.

Before you eat anything, try to listen to your stomach, not your head. If your stomach is growling or pinching, you're really hungry. If it isn't, then you just want to eat.

Remember, you can indulge sometimes, too. If you're craving corn chips, go for it! But grab out a handful and put it into a bowl, do NOT eat straight from the bag!

It's very important to learn portion control. You can't eat unlimited amounts of almost any food without gaining weight. Yes, you can eat to your heart's content on cucumbers or lettuce, but most foods need to be limited.

In the next chapter, I'm going to make a list of foods you can eat whenever you're hungry, including foods that you can have in practically unlimited quantities.

We'll also look at some food substitutions you can use to satisfy cravings for higher-fat foods. While this won't always work, sometimes it does.

Weight Loss Tips for the Struggling Dieter

Whenever you can cut calories with substitutions, it's a great thing!

WHAT ARE POWER FOODS?

This chapter is all about telling you what you can safely eat. We're going to talk about foods you should eat whenever you're having a craving for something fattening, stuff you can substitute for the bad stuff.

The main thing is to keep your fridge and cabinets stocked with plenty of foods you can eat in unlimited or substantial quantities.

First, let's talk about some things you can eat in unlimited quantities. These are foods that, if you eat them until you feel like you're going to puke, you still shouldn't fear gaining any weight!

These are also foods that contain vitamins, minerals, and other essential elements.

They are foods you can feel good about eating, and you don't have to feel guilty, even if you overeat them. They are also rich in antioxidants and perhaps other important elements that scientists haven't even discovered, yet!

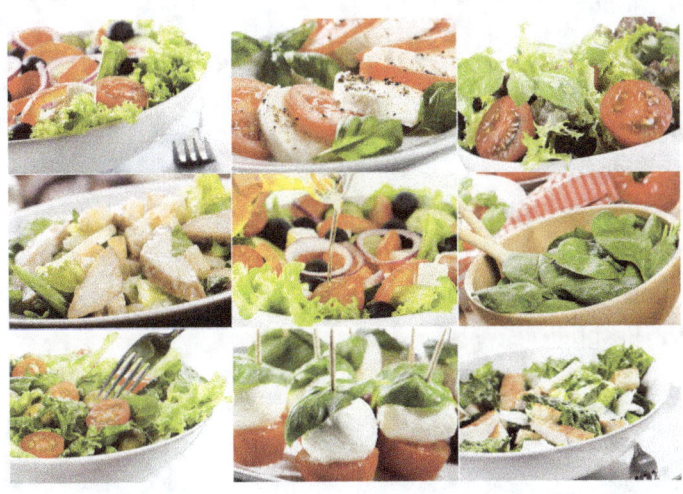

Weight Loss Tips for the Struggling Dieter

Foods to eat in unlimited quantities:

- ❖ Apples
- ❖ Asparagus
- ❖ Beets
- ❖ Blueberries
- ❖ Cabbage
- ❖ Cantaloupe
- ❖ Carrots
- ❖ Cauliflower
- ❖ Celery
- ❖ Cranberries
- ❖ Cucumbers
- ❖ Dill Pickles (Kosher or Hamburger Dill)
- ❖ Fresh Herbs or Dried
- ❖ Garlic
- ❖ Grapefruit
- ❖ Green Beans
- ❖ Greens (All Types)
- ❖ Honeydew Melons
- ❖ Lemons and Limes
- ❖ Lettuce
- ❖ Mangoes
- ❖ Mushrooms
- ❖ Onions
- ❖ Papayas
- ❖ Peaches
- ❖ Peppers (All Kinds)
- ❖ Pineapple
- ❖ Radishes
- ❖ Raspberries
- ❖ Spinach
- ❖ Strawberries
- ❖ Tangerines
- ❖ Tomatoes

  - ❖ Turnips
  - ❖ Watermelon
  - ❖ Zucchini

You can combine these ingredients into delicious recipes that taste great, too. This will help keep you motivated. The better tasting the food is that you're eating; the more likely it is you will stick to the system.

These ingredients can work very well together. For example, you could take some of the vegetables like tomatoes, cabbage, onions, carrots, zucchini, celery, and green beans and make a very nice soup.

You could also use unlimited fresh herbs or dried herbs to flavor it.

You could make a nice fruit salad using various fruits, flavorings, and herbs.

Mint and cilantro both go very well with many different types of fruits, and lemon or limejuice with a touch of salt can make a sweet fruit salad a bit more savory.

Lemon juice can also be used on its own with herbs, or blended with fruit to make a dressing for salads.

A salad of spinach and sliced mushrooms tastes amazing with vinaigrette of raspberries, cranberries, or strawberries with lemon juice, red wine vinegar, salt, and pepper.

Experiment with using these ingredients to make various recipes. You can also add small amounts of foods that aren't on the list, comprising a recipe mostly of these items and using other foods as flavorings.

For example, you could make a soup using these vegetables and using a small amount of boneless, skinless chicken breast to flavor it and add protein. Or you could make a delicious salsa with tomatoes, onions, jalapeno peppers, cilantro, and lime juice, and then serve it over lettuce with a 1 cup of black beans.

The combinations are practically endless, especially when you start using foods that you can't have in unlimited quantities to bring flavors together.

Now you need to know some flavorings you can use in unlimited quantities. Some condiments are high in sugar or fat, and you should avoid these for the most part. You can enjoy small quantities of them, but it's best to limit them.

Flavorings to enjoy in unlimited quantities:

- ❖ Mustard
- ❖ Vinegar (All Types)
- ❖ Spices (No Sugar, No or Low Sodium)
- ❖ Herbs
- ❖ Lemon Juice
- ❖ Lime Juice

Make sure the flavorings you buy do not contain MSG. There are many seasonings on the market that do. The salt replacement Accent, in fact, IS monosodium glutamate; so avoid this one at all costs! Look for flavorings that contain as little sodium as possible, but you don't have to avoid it completely.

Next, let's look at some various types of proteins you can add to the unlimited foods to bring a meal together and make it more filling.

You should limit these foods to smaller servings, but you should make sure to use some of these every day.

Proteins to enjoy in smaller quantities:

- ❖ Boneless, Skinless Chicken Breast
- ❖ Turkey Breast
- ❖ Most Types of Fish
- ❖ Lean Beef
- ❖ Beans (All Types)
- ❖ Other Lean Meats
- ❖ Tofu
- ❖ Nuts

Lean meats, beans, nuts, and tofu are filling. They also provide nutrients like iron that are essential for a healthy body. They should be used more as a flavoring for other foods than a major part of the meal, especially when trying to lose weight.

Vegetarians can obviously leave meat out entirely, opting for vegetable-based protein sources. There is a lot of controversy about whether soy-based products like tofu are good for you or not, but I personally use it in small quantities.

Flavorings to enjoy in smaller quantities:

- ❖ Salt
- ❖ Ketchup (Preferably Sugar-Free)
- ❖ Olive Oil (Limit Carefully)
- ❖ Agaves Nectar (Liquid Sweetener, Natural, Won't Spike Blood Sugar)
- ❖ Soy Sauce (High In Sodium, So Limit)

You shouldn't eliminate salt from your diet completely, as your body does need a bit of salt to run properly. But these should be limited as much as possible.

Olive oil is one of the healthiest oils you can use. Studies have shown that people who consume around two tablespoons of olive oil daily for one week show less oxidation of LDL cholesterol, as well as higher levels of antioxidants in their blood.

Olive oil can help protect against ulcers and gastritis. It may help prevent colon cancer. It contains vitamin # and phenols. In short, it is probably the best fat you can possibly consume.

As with nearly anything, it should be consumed in limited quantities. It is still very high in calories, and of course, is pure fat. Eating enough of it will cause you to gain weight, but it should still be used in small amounts because of its protective benefits.

Agave nectar is a natural sweetener that comes from a type of cactus.

It tastes very sweet, but it won't spike your blood sugar like process sugar, honey, syrup, and other sweeteners. It's also considered much safer than aspartame and other chemical sweeteners.

Wendy Chin

The Importance of Moderation

Now that we've talked about the foods you should eat, let's talk about the foods you should avoid whenever possible.

These are foods that can really mess up your weight loss efforts, and it's best to avoid most of them completely, or carefully restrict them.

For the most part, you should feel free to enjoy the foods you love, just in lesser quantities. Unfortunately, many of the foods you love will contain these "forbidden foods".

Because I believe in indulging on occasion in order to keep yourself happily sticking to your weight loss plan, I don't exactly advocate cutting these foods out completely.

What I do suggest is that you limit these foods very carefully, indulging in them only when you are having a desperate craving for them and you feel like you might go overboard and binge if you don't have them at that moment.

Sugar

Sugar, specifically white sugar, is a very bad substance. I highly recommend avoiding it as much as possible.

While it's unrealistic to expect you to never eat anything that contains white sugar again, you should try to avoid it whenever possible.

Sugar is believed to be a major instigator of diabetes. It causes blood sugar levels to rise rapidly, and then they can cause an over-production of insulin.

When you have too much insulin in your body, it can cause your cells to hold on to fat. It can also cause your liver to create extra fat from the calories you consume.

Excess insulin can cause blood clots that lead to stroke and heart attack, raise LDL (bad) cholesterol levels, and can cause plaque to form in the arteries. It can also raise your blood pressure by causing your kidneys to retain salt.

If your body continuously produces too much insulin, it can lead to a condition known as insulin resistance. Insulin resistance can lead to severe obesity, and it can make it extremely difficult to lose weight.

Sugar is one of the worst substances you can eat, and I highly recommend avoiding it.

Remember, sugar isn't found only in cookies, cakes, and sodas. It can be found hiding in places you wouldn't expect it. Sugar is often found in salad dressings, gravies, sauces, condiments, cereal, and even bread and breaded meats!

White Flour

White flour is another substance that causes blood sugar levels to rise very rapidly. White flour is used in most baked products, as well as various types of breading, and even as a thickener in many sauces.

Like sugar, it is a substance that causes very severe blood sugar spikes, which can then lead to crashes. White flour is one of the worst culprits, so I highly recommend avoiding it as much as possible.

Wendy Chin

White flour is found in so many different things, it will be difficult to avoid them all. If you're a huge fan of baked goods, it will be almost impossible to avoid it altogether.

If you aren't going to cut out white flour completely, I urge you to cut down sharply on your consumption of it. White flour is one of the worst things you can consume, and second only to sugar, in my opinion.

Switch to whole grain products whenever possible. Limit white flour products, and only indulge in them on rare occasions. I like to have cake on birthdays, but for the most part I try to avoid white flour completely.

Potatoes

I know potatoes are delicious. In fact, they are one of my favorite foods. But they spike blood sugar. Potatoes are very high in carbohydrates, and they are "bad carbs" – the kind that raise blood sugar very quickly.

Sweet potatoes, on the other hand, don't raise blood sugar so quickly. Even though they are technically "sweet", they just don't have quite such an extreme effect on blood sugar levels.

If you're going to eat potatoes, I do suggest eating sweet potatoes rather than other types of potatoes. Not only will they not spike your blood sugar, but sweet potatoes are also very high in vitamins, while white potatoes have very little nutritional value.

White Rice

White rice is another major cause of blood sugar spikes. It is consumed around the world, and people believe that because

Asian people eat a lot of white rice and seem to be so thin and healthy, that white rice must be healthy.

The problem is, they aren't looking at the other factors involved in the health of so many Asians. Asians tend to get a lot more exercise than Western people.

They eat far less meat and junk food. They consume a lot more fresh fruits and vegetables. And they eat a lot of healthy seafood.

Because white rice causes these extreme blood sugar spikes, you should substitute brown rice for white whenever possible. The blood sugar spikes are mitigated by the fiber, which is left intact on the outside of the grains in brown rice.

In most cases, high-fiber ingredients won't cause the type of blood sugar spikes seen in their refined counterparts.

There aren't a whole lot of foods that I would suggest avoiding completely. Basically, if a food has little or no nutritional value, it's not worth eating and should be avoided.

You can indulge in these foods on occasion, but I would keep it to no more often than once per week. That doesn't mean you can have white rice once per week, potatoes once per week, sugar once per week, and white flour once per week! It means you should have ONE item per week that contains one or more of these items.

And remember to control your portion. Just because you can have these items only once per week does not mean you should eat an entire cake at one sitting!

Wendy Chin

SOME GREAT WEIGHT LOSS TIPS

You should eat when you're hungry. It's that simple. The trick is in learning how to know when you're actually hungry, and when you want to eat because you are tired, bored, stressed out, or just craving food.

This is actually harder than it sounds for many people. After years, perhaps decades of eating for the wrong reasons, you may have to train your body to recognize hunger again.

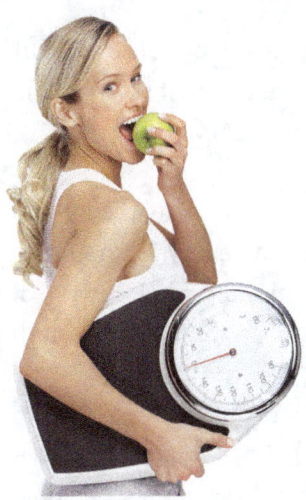

Hunger usually involves stomach pinches, pains, or growling. If your stomach isn't growling, you're probably not really hungry. But this isn't always indicative of hunger.

Sometimes you may feel food moving around in your stomach from your last meal, and this may mimic very closely the feeling you have when you're hungry.

Before you rush to eat after your stomach starts growling, wait just a little while to see if the growling subsides. If it doesn't go away in

10-15 minutes, or if you feel weak or jittery, it's probably true hunger. If the growling goes away, it might have been the feeling of food being digested.

I suggest eating several smaller meals per day rather than 3 large ones. When you eat smaller meals, you can help boost your metabolism. The more often your body is consuming food, the faster your metabolism will become.

You see, your body will digest food slowly to make the energy it gets from food and the full feeling last as long as possible if it thinks it isn't getting enough food.

When you're consuming a lot of food regularly, it realizes that there is an abundance of food, and it will respond by digesting food quickly and giving you plenty of energy.

I don't recommend waiting a certain amount of time between meals. Ideally you'll be eating every 2-4 hours, just small amounts, but you may need to eat an hour after a meal, of you may not feel hungry for 4-5 hours. Just learn to listen to your body's own hunger signals.

You should aim for eating smaller, almost snack-sized meals about 4-6 times per day. Eating three meals per day will mean you're eating more at each meal.

This can spike your blood sugar and cause you to crash, leading to cravings when you're not actually hungry.

Eating a lot at one meal can also cause you to experience something commonly known as "food coma". This is mostly caused by eating a large amount of food at one time, especially foods that are high in refined carbohydrates.

It takes a lot of energy to digest food. It can be especially taxing when your blood sugar spikes and crashes. This causes energy to be diverted from other systemic functions, causing your brain to feel "foggy", and the rest of your body to feel weak and tired.

While the tryptophan in turkey can indeed cause sleepiness, it is probably mostly the "food coma" effect that causes you to feel so tired and sluggish after a holiday meal. Thanksgiving and other holiday meals are usually very high in carbohydrates and sugar, and people tend to overeat at these meals.

The same thing can happen to you anytime you eat a large meal, especially one that is high in refined carbohydrates.

When you eat smaller, lighter meals, you will feel energized after eating, rather than tired and run-down.

Remember, the primary goal of eating smaller meals throughout the day is to keep your metabolism charged up. The higher your metabolism, the faster the weight will melt off.

SIMPLE WEIGHT LOSS STRATEGIES

Getting exercise is very important in order to increase your metabolism and help you burn fat.

You don't have to bench press 250 pounds or run the Boston Marathon to get exercise. There are some very simple, easy, and fun ways to get exercise!

And don't tell me you don't have enough time to exercise! There are opportunities to get exercise all around you. All you have to do is take them!

We're going to look at some ways you can work exercise into your day, no matter how busy you are. Let's face it, almost everyone is busy.

We all have things like school, work, and children to deal with. Most of us don't have nearly as much time as we'd like to complete our daily tasks, must less to exercise and get any entertainment! But there are ways to work exercise into your normal day!

In additional to pursuing activities you may really enjoy such as bowling, tennis, swimming, hiking, and other physical activities that might be enjoyable, you can use these tips to make sure you get more exercise every day.

Walk More

Take the stairs whenever you can. Elevators are helpful if you have many flights to ascend, or if you're carrying packages, or if you have small children with you, or if you're already extremely exhausted or injured. But you should take the stairs whenever it is feasible.Start looking for ways to get more walking into your day. It

Wendy Chin

has been said that it takes at least 20-30 minutes of aerobic exercise at a time to have a benefit, but recent studies have shown that may not be true.

One study revealed that people who exercised a total of 20-30 minutes each day in increments of just a few minutes at a time still experienced the same cardiac benefit as those who exercised for 20-30 minutes at one time.

Plus, it doesn't make a difference to how many calories are burned whether you break it up or do it all at once. You will also benefit from increased muscle, and muscle tissue burns a lot more energy than fat tissue!

Television Workouts

Most people watch a lot of television. The average American watches 28 hours of television per week, about 4 hours every day! That's a lot of time wasted in front of the tube!

You can put that time to good use by exercising while you are watching television. There are plenty of exercises you can do in front of the TV.

- ❖ Walking on a treadmill
- ❖ Riding an exercise bike
- ❖ Sit-ups and crunches
- ❖ Lifting weights
- ❖ Toe touches
- ❖ Pushups
- ❖ Leg lifts
- ❖ Walking in place
- ❖ Bouncing on a rebounder (mini trampoline)
- ❖ Using a stair stepper

These are all fun, healthy, and not very disruptive of your television watching. You can do many of these exercises while reading a book or magazine, catching up on the local news in the newspaper, or listening to music, too.

Office Workouts

There are plenty of things you can do at your desk while you're at work or school, too. Students and office workers often find that they don't get enough exercise, because they spend most of their day sitting down. They may have to walk from class to class or run errands, but for the most part, they are very sedentary all day.

This is where it comes in handy to perform exercises that can be done while sitting at a desk. While it won't exactly be aerobic exercise, it will help you tone your muscles. Not only will you look better, but remember, muscle burns more calories than fat!

Stomach crunches will help you get your stomach muscles toned. Simply suck in and hold your stomach muscles tight and taught for several seconds, then release. Perform this action continually throughout the day whenever you think about it.

You can also walk around doing this during the day. You'll be toning and building your abdominal muscles while also sucking in and making your belly look flatter!

You can pull your toes upwards and stretch your calf muscles. Just point your toes up toward your knees as far as you can without it becoming painful, hold for a few seconds, and release. Repeat this several times. This can also help prevent blood clots, which are more common in sedentary individuals.

Your bottom may also be somewhat flabby. If so, you can clench your gluteus maximus muscles tightly while sitting in your desk.

Wendy Chin

Hold briefly, and then release. This will help build and tighten your buttocks.

These types of exercises will also work for other parts of your body, including your back, biceps, triceps, forearms, and thighs. Just clench your muscles, hold briefly, and release.

Remember to be careful not to injure yourself. Too much of a good thing is not good. Don't stretch your muscles until they are painful. A slight discomfort is completely normal, but pain is not. Never work out until you feel pain!

I hope you can see how easy it is to get exercise. You can find time here and there, whenever and wherever you can. Any exercise is better than no exercise at all!

How to Maintain Your Weight

Once you've lost the weight, you need to learn how to keep it off. Most people do gain the weight back after they lose it, because they go right back to their old habits.

As you get closer to your goal weight, you will need to start easing into the lifestyle that you will continue for the rest of your life.

You will need to remember to keep cutting out the biggest sources of blood sugar spikes, including sugar, white flour, white rice, and potatoes. You will need to continue consuming plenty of fresh fruits and vegetables, healthy seafood, and other lean proteins. And you will need to continue getting some exercise.

Always remember that if you don't continue the lifestyle, you are doomed to repeat everything you've just been through.

You'll have to deal with the pain of being overweight, the embarrassment you feel when you go out in public, the difficulty losing the weight, the aches, pains, and discomfort of being overweight, and all of those other issues.

That's something you don't ever want to have to go through again, right?

Never let go of the things you're feeling right now. Never forget the struggle. Never forget the pain. Never, ever forget.

Once you let go, once you get past it and you move on, you cannot forget. If you allow yourself to forget what it was like, you'll be back on that road to obesity before you know it.

Wendy Chin

It's a good idea to keep a lot of photos of yourself before you lost the weight. Keep a journal of how difficult your dieting is. Write notes in it about how horrible you feel, how embarrassed you are, how your life is miserable. Keep all of this together and look at it regularly.

Yes, it will be painful to dredge up those memories of when you were so unhealthy, but it will help you stay healthy.

The emotional pain you feel will be nothing compared to what your friends and family would feel if they lost you because you had a heart attack or stroke due to obesity, or the pain you would feel if you gained all of the weight back.

Keep eating healthily. Keep exercising. Keep living the healthiest life possible.

SOME GREAT WORKOUT & MUSCLE BUILDING TIPS

Let's take a look at just some of the most common exercises and routines so you better understand the different techniques used within weight training and overall fitness.

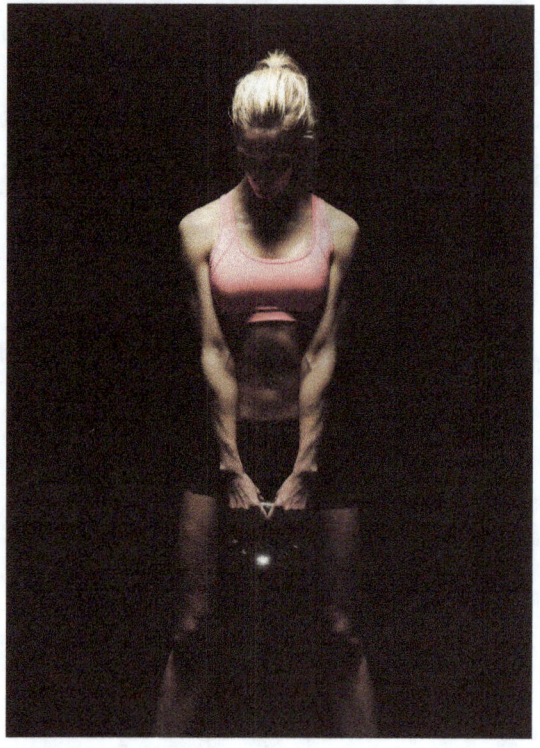

Here are a few of the more common ones:

Dumbbell Bench Press

Sit on the edge of a flat bench with the dumbbells resting on your knees. In one smooth motion, roll onto your back and bring the dumbbells up to a position slightly outside and above your shoulders. Your palms should be facing forwards.

Bend your elbows at a ninety-degree angle with your upper arms parallel to the ground. Press the weights up over your chest in a triangular motion until they meet above the centerline of your body.

As you lift, concentrate on keeping the weights balanced and under control.

Follow the same path downward.

Standing Military Press

For this exercise, you will use a barbell. Stand with your legs about shoulder width apart and lift the barbell to your chest. Lock your legs and hips and keep your elbows in slightly under the bar. Press the bar to arm's length over your head.

Lower the bell to your upper chest or your chin depending on which is more comfortable for you.

This exercise can also be performed with dumbbells or seated on a weight bench.

Lying Tricep Push

Sit on a flat bench holding a curl bar with an overhand grip. Lie back so that the top of your head is even with the end of the weight bench. As you are lying back, extend your arms over your head so that the bar is directly over your eyes.

Keep your elbows tight and your upper arms stationary throughout the exercise.

The biggest key to this exercise is keeping your upper arms in a fixed position.

Slowly lower the bar until it almost touches your forehead. Press the bar back up in a slow, sweeping arc-like motion. At the finish, lock your elbows completely.

Side Lateral Dumbbell Raise

Stand upright with your feet shoulder width apart and your arms at your side. Hold a dumbbell in each hand with your palms turned toward your body.

Keep your arms straight and lift the weights out and up to the sides until they are slightly higher than shoulder level.

Then slowly lower them back down to your side again.

Keep your palms turned downward as you lift the dumbbells so that your shoulders rather than your biceps do the work.

Make sure you are lifting the dumbbells up rather than swinging them up. Don't lean forward while doing this either or you risk injury to your back.

Preacher Curls

This exercise is best done with a special preacher curl bench, but you can do this without it with a little modification.

Sit at the end of the weight bench, and place something such as a firm pillow or a few pillows under your armpits on your lap. Hold the curl bar in your hands with palms facing upward.

Don't hunch over the pillow, sit as straight as you can.

Wendy Chin

Using a shoulder width grip, grasp the bar in both hands. Curl the bar upward in an arc. Be careful not to swing or rock to get the bar moving. You need to be using your muscles to lift the weight, not momentum. The goal of this exercise is to work the biceps.

Bring the bar up to your chin keeping in mind that the resistance is greatest during the beginning of the lift. Lower the bar slowly working the muscle on the way down as well.

You can also do this with dumbbells or work one arm at a time.

Seated Dumbbell Curl

Sit at the end of a bench with your feet firmly on the floor. Keep your back straight and your head up. Start with the dumbbells at arm's length with your palms facing in. Curl the weight up and twist your wrist once they pass your thighs.

Squeeze your biceps at the top and then slowly lower the weight.

Do not swing the dumbbells down; lower them as you are working those muscles! You can do this standing, but the seated position prevents bad form.

One-Arm Dumbbell Row

Start with your right foot flat on the floor and your left knee resting on a flat bench.

Lean forward so that you're supporting the weight of your upper body with your left arm on the bench. Your back should be flat and almost parallel with the floor.

Reach down and pick up a dumbbell with your right hand. Your left arm should be locked at the elbow so it will support the weight of your upper body.

Before starting, look straight ahead instead of at the floor so you can keep your back straight. Tighten your abs to keep your body from turning to the side as you lift the dumbbell.

Concentrate on pulling your elbow back as far as it can go. The dumbbell should end up roughly parallel with your torso.

After you've rowed the dumbbell up as far as you can slowly lower it back to the starting position. Switch arms after one set.

Dumbbell Shrugs

Stand straight up with your feet at shoulder width. Hold two dumbbells with your arms hanging at your sides.

Droop your shoulders down as far as possible. Raise your shoulders up as far as you can go then slowly return to the starting position.

You can also rotate your shoulders by going up in a circular motion from front to back and then back down again. This can also be done holding a barbell.

Standing Calf Raises

This can be done with a specific machine found in a gym, or adapted for use without the machine. Stand up against a wall with your body facing the wall and your palms down on the wall and your feet flat on the floor.

Keep your body straight and slowly lift up your heels until you are standing on the tips of your toes. Hold the contraction briefly then slowly return to the starting position with your feet flat on the floor.

Crunches

Wendy Chin

Lie flat on your back with your feet flat on the ground, or resting on a bench with your knees bent at a 90 degree angle. If you are resting your feet on a bench, place them three to four inches apart and point your toes inward so they touch.

Place your hands lightly on either side of your head keeping your elbows in. Don't lock your fingers behind your head! Push the small of your back down in the floor to isolate your abdominal muscles. Begin to roll your shoulders off the floor.

Continue to push down as hard as you can with your lower back.

Your shoulders should come up off the floor only about four inches, and your lower back should remain on the floor. Focus on slow, controlled movement - don't cheat yourself by using momentum!

Dumbbell Hammer Curls

With a dumbbell in each hand, stand with your arms hanging at your sides, and palms are facing each other. Keep your elbows locked into your sides. Your upper body and elbows should remain in the same place during the whole lift.

Keep your palms facing each other, curl the weight in your right hand up in a semi-circle toward your right shoulder. Squeeze the biceps hard at the top of the lift and then slowly lower.

Do not turn your wrists during this lift! You can also do one arm at a time and/or alternate.

Incline Dumbbell Press

Sit on the edge of an incline bench set at about a 45-degree angle. Pick up a dumbbell in each hand and place them on your thighs.

Then, one at a time, raise them up to your shoulder level while you press your back and shoulders firmly against the bench.

Press the weights back up to a point over your upper chest, with your palms facing forward. Lower the weights slowly. Inhale as you lower the weights and exhale as you lift.

Barbell Squat

Rest a barbell on the upper portion of your back, not your neck. Firmly grip the bar with your hands almost twice your shoulder width apart.

Position your feet about shoulder width apart and your toes should be pointing just a little outward with your knees in the same direction.

Keep your back as straight as possible and your chin up, bend your knees and slowly lower your hips straight down until your thighs are parallel to the floor. Once you reach the bottom position, press the weight up back to the starting position.

Don't lean over or curve your back forward! You can use a belt to help reduce the chance of lower back injury. You can put your heels on a 1 inch block to further work the quads. You can also use a wider stance to work the inner quads even more.

Upright Barbell Row

Stand upright and grasp a barbell with your hands about shoulder width apart. Let the bar hang straight down in front of you. Keep your body and wrists straight. Pull the bar straight up towards your chin, keeping it close to your body.

Concentrate on either pulling with your traps or the front of your shoulders, depending on what you want to work most. Lower slowly to the starting position. Don't cheat by leaning forward or backward. Don't swing!

Front Dumbbell Raise

Stand with a dumbbell in each hand, palms facing backward. Your feet should be about shoulder width apart. Maintain a slight bend in your elbows throughout the exercise so that your arms are straight, but not quite locked.

Lift the weight in your left hand in front of you in a wide arc until it is slightly higher than shoulder height.

With a smooth, controlled motion, lower the weight while simultaneously lifting the weight in your right hand, so that both arms are in motion at the same time.

Do not cheat by swinging or leaning backwards! This lift can also be done with two dumbbells at the same time or a barbell.

Stiff Leg Barbell

Place a barbell on your shoulders. Keep your head up and your back completely straight.

Bend at your waist with your legs locked, until your upper body is parallel to the floor.

Return slowly to the upper position. This can also be done with your knees slightly bent.

One Leg Barbell Squat

Use a 12 to 18 inch box or bench for this exercise - the higher the box, the more difficult the exercise. Place a barbell behind your head at the base of your neck. Grasp the barbell with both hands with a wider than shoulder width grip.

Stand approximately 2 to 3 feet from the box and turn so that the box is directly behind you. Reach one foot back and place your toe on the box.

Keep your opposite foot flat on the floor and point your toes forward. Stand up straight. Keep your back tight and your chest out throughout the entire exercise.

Keep your head and neck in line with your torso so that you are looking forward. Your shoulders should be directly over your front foot.

Keeping your front foot flat on the floor, sit your hips back (like you are going to sit in a chair), bend your knee (of your front leg), and lean forward slightly at the waist.

Lower your body in a controlled fashion until your thigh (of your front leg) is parallel to the ground.

If you have difficulty lowering yourself down this far, lower yourself until the knee of your front leg is bent 90 degrees.

At this point, your knee should be directly over your toe, your hips should be sitting back, and your chest should be directly over the middle of your thigh.

Now, leading with your head and chest, raise yourself by pushing your hips slightly forward and up toward the ceiling, and straightening your leg. Return to the starting position.

Wendy Chin

At this point, your shoulders should be directly over front foot.

Lunges

Place a barbell on your upper back. Lift your chest up and look straight ahead. Position your right leg forward in a long stride.

Your foot should be far enough in front of you so that when you bend your right knee, your thigh and lower leg form a right angle.

Slowly bend your knees, lowering your hips so your rear knee just clears the floor. Pause briefly in this position, then slowly straighten your legs and raise your body back up to a standing position.

Complete a full set, then switch legs and repeat, or alternate legs for each rep.

Make sure your knee does not travel past your toes in the down position! This can also be done with dumbbells in each hand instead of using a barbell.

Barbell Tricep Extension

Hold a barbell with hands a little closer together than shoulder width. Lie on an incline bench and position your head at the top.

Press bar overhead to arm's length. Lower the bar in a semicircular motion behind your head until your forearms touch your biceps.

Keep your upper arms close to your head. Return to the starting position. This can also be done with straight bar, 2 dumbbells, seated or standing or with 2 dumbbells and your palms facing in.

Notes:

With any workout, you need to start out with some warm up exercises. This can be simple stretching as you get your body ready to work. A warm-up session prior to working out can not only help get your body ready for exercise, but your mind will get prepared as well.

You should also have an appropriate cool down period after you are done working out.

This will reduce the possibility of delayed muscle soreness and will help quell the adrenaline that has been building in your system as a result of the workout. This can also be simple stretching exercises and deep breathing.

Again, it's important to start out slow and not push yourself beyond your limits.

ABOUT THE AUTHOR

One other thing Wendy advises in her weight loss journey was to Increase how much yard work you have outdoors by starting a garden. Gardening burns a few hundred calories in only an hour, depending on the type of work you do. Between clearing out a space, tilling, planting seeds or plants, pruning, watering, and other things you do to keep a garden looking beautiful, you will be out there at least a few days a week. Now is the perfect time to start that garden you have always wanted, while also getting more physical activity for losing or maintaining your weight. Bonus? Plant vegetables and eat healthier from the fruits of that labor. Grab a copy of Wendy's book Weight Loss Tips for the Struggling Dieter.

www.ingramcontent.com/pod-product-compliance
Lightning Source LLC
Chambersburg PA
CBHW071131280526
45787CB00003B/1247